LITTLE SHOTS
FOR LITTLE TOTS

WRITTEN BY BRANDY ROY
ILLUSTRATED BY MANDY MORREALE

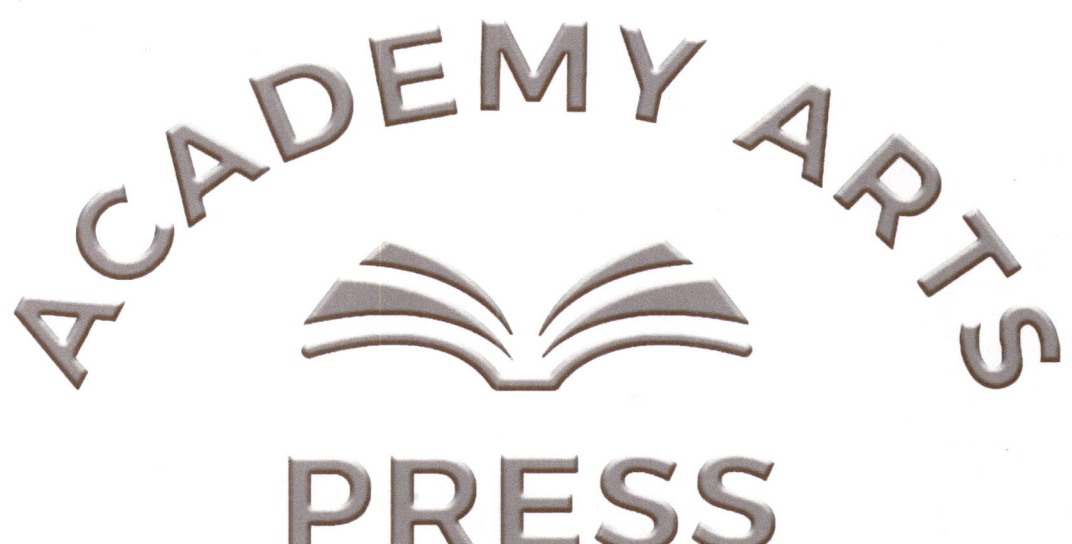

ACADEMY ARTS
PRESS

WWW.ACADEMYARTSPRESS.COM

@T1DTODDLER

Hello, my name is Ryder.
What is your name?
We both have diabetes.
So we are both the same.

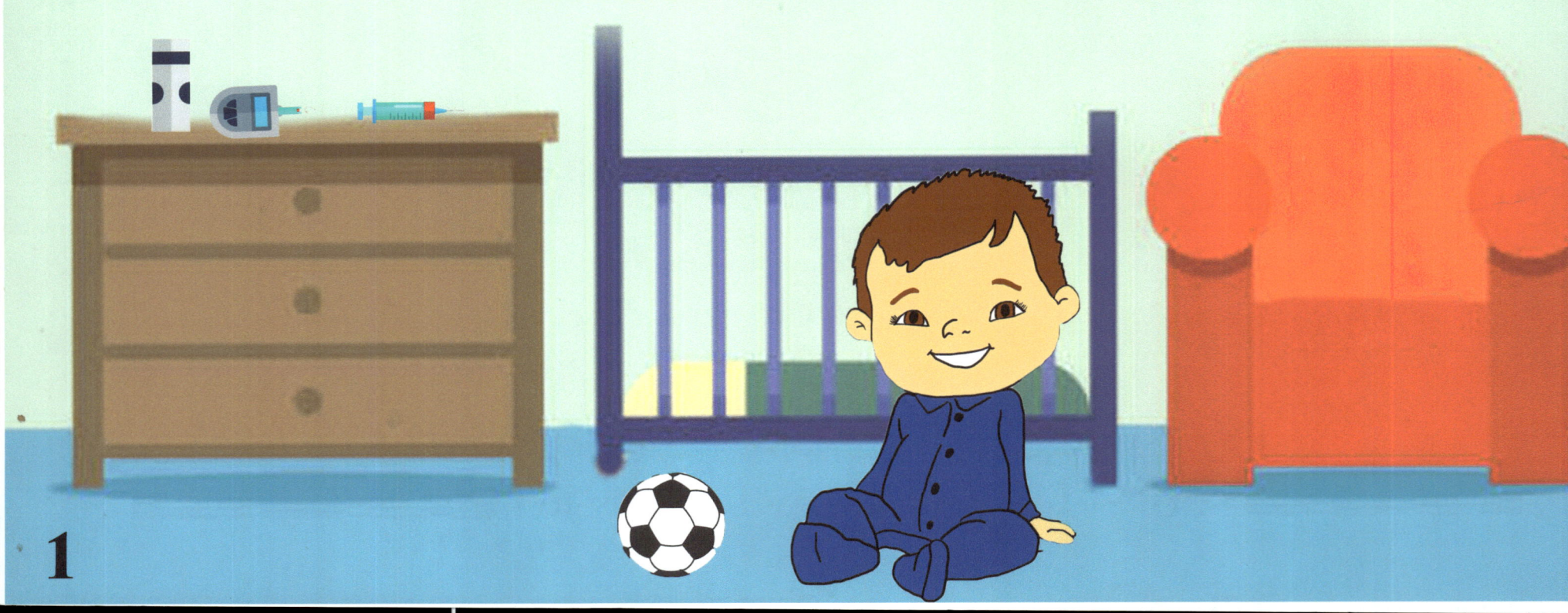

IF YOU'RE READING THIS
THEN WELCOME TO THE CLUB.
IT'S FULL OF WARRIORS JUST LIKE YOU
WHO LEARN TO NOT GIVE UP!

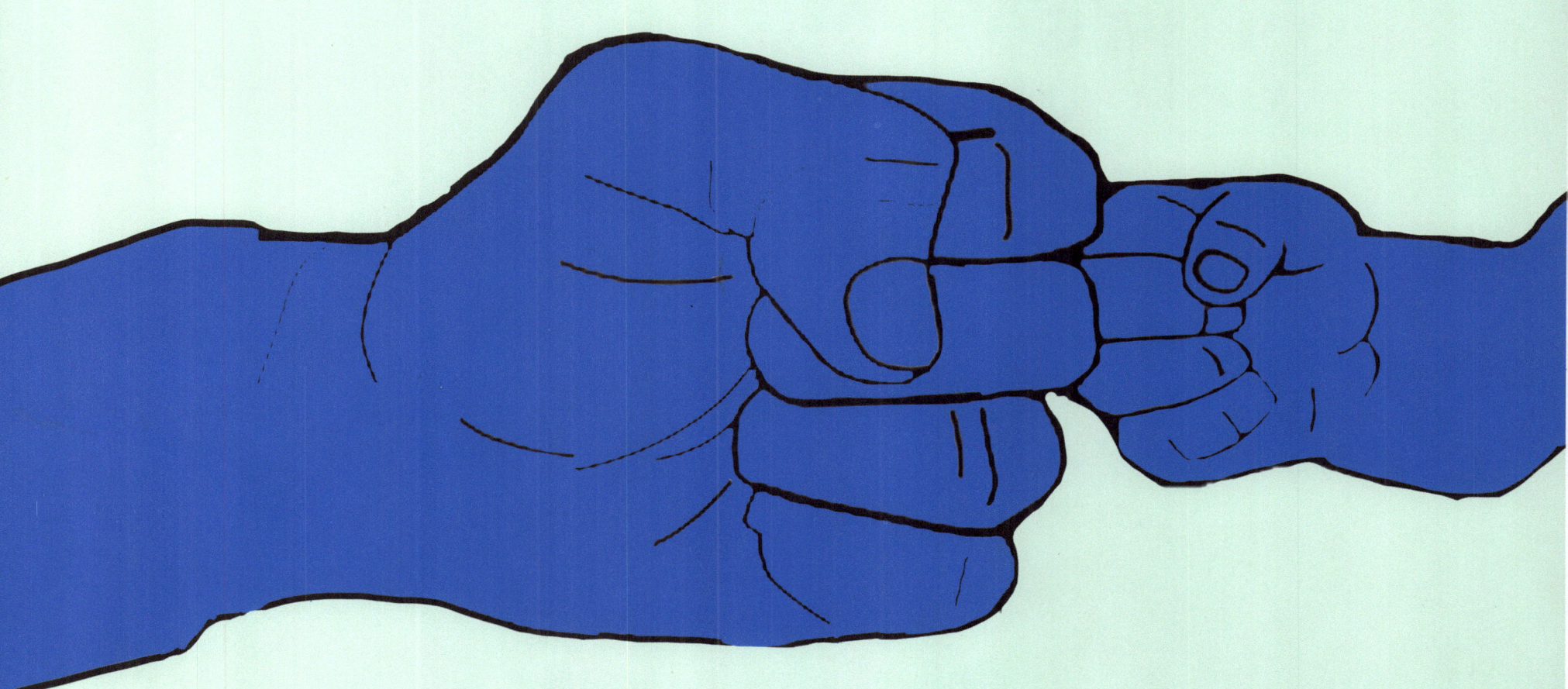

WELCOME EVERY MOMENT.
THE GOOD ONES
AND THE BAD.
AND YOU DON'T
HAVE TO WORRY,
YOU'VE GOT YOUR
MOM AND DAD.

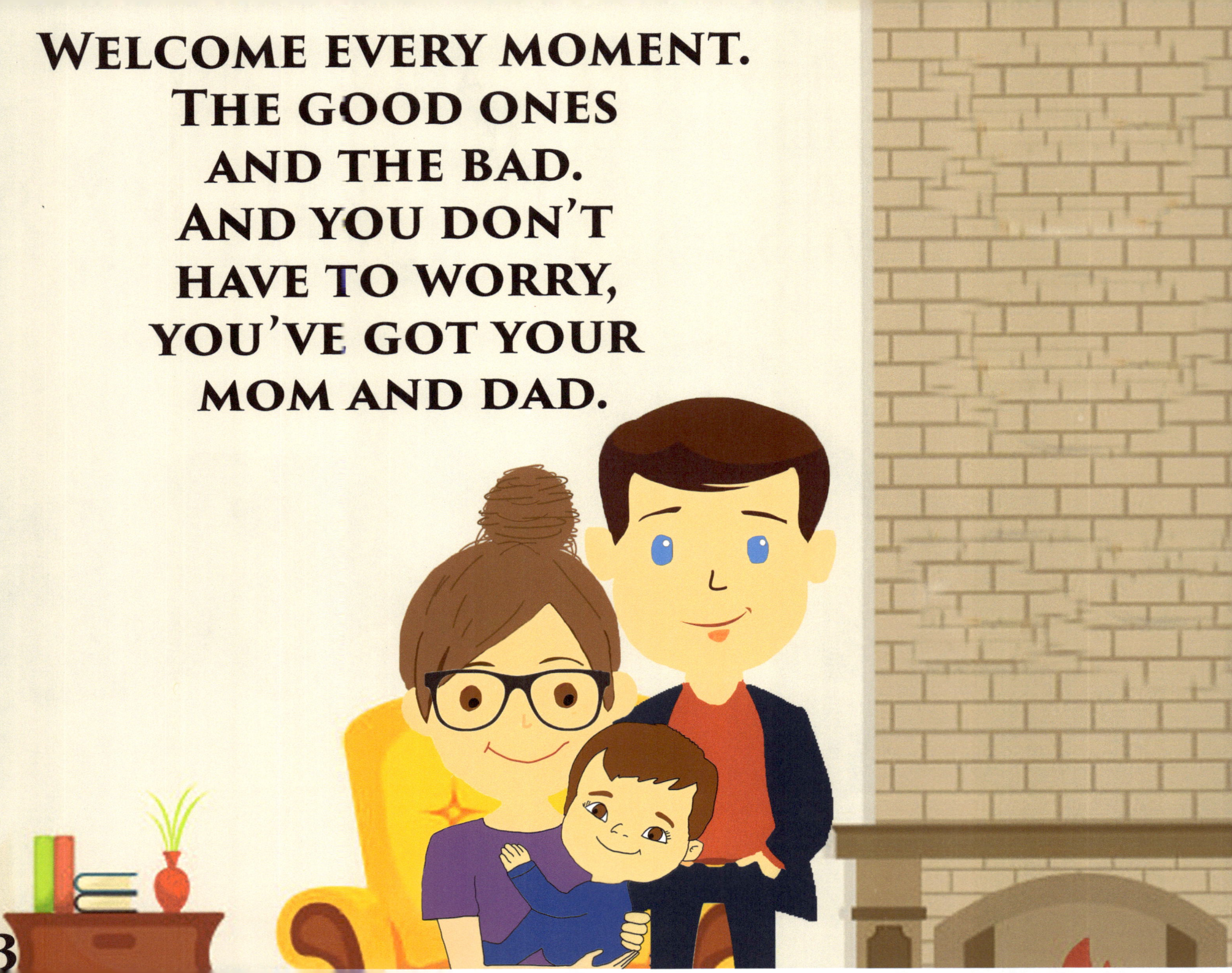

3

TOGETHER YOU'LL GET THROUGH THIS.
AS A FAMILY.
ALONG WITH MANY OTHERS, WE'LL FIGHT DIABETES.

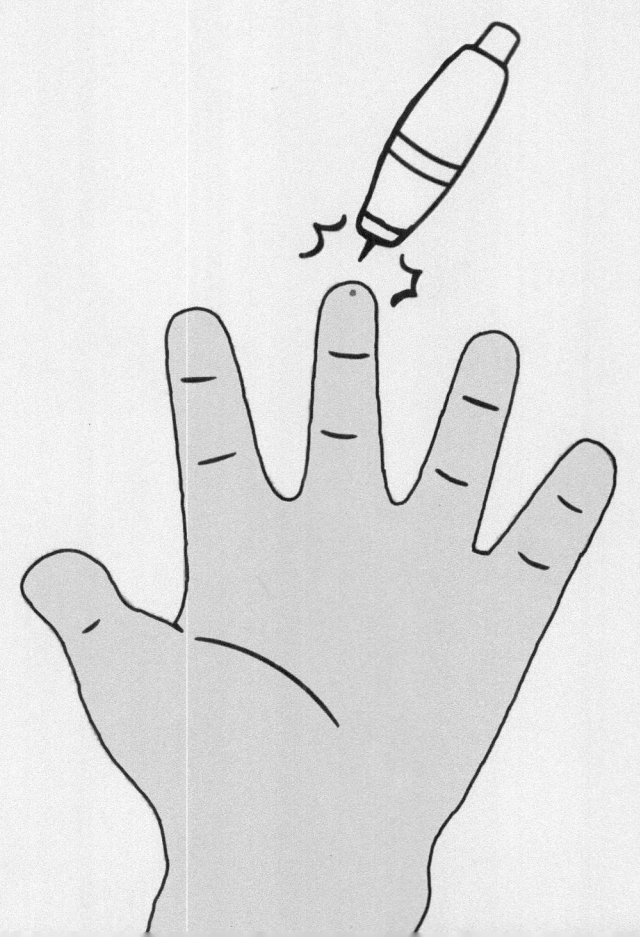

FIRST THERE WERE THE SIGNS.
LOST WEIGHT AND
HAVING TO PEE.
MOODY AND NOT HUNGRY,
BUT I SURE WAS THIRSTY.

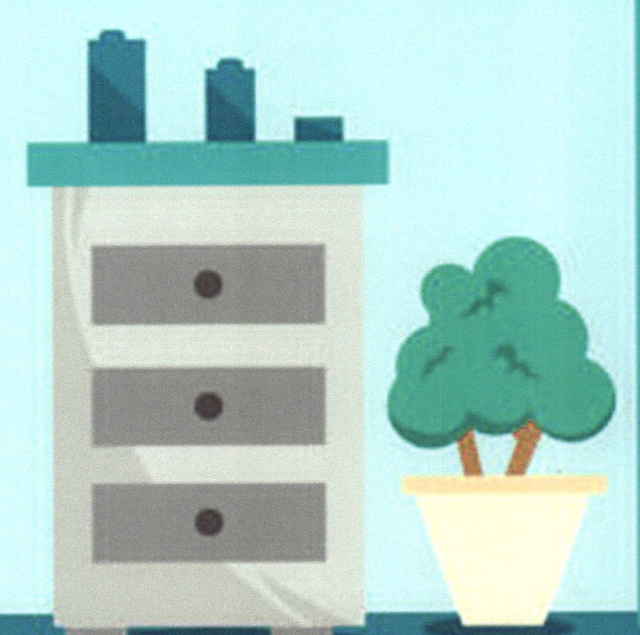

THEN THERE WERE THE DOCTORS,
THE NEEDLES AND THE TESTS.
IT TOOK SOME TIME
TO FIGURE OUT
I WASN'T AT MY BEST.

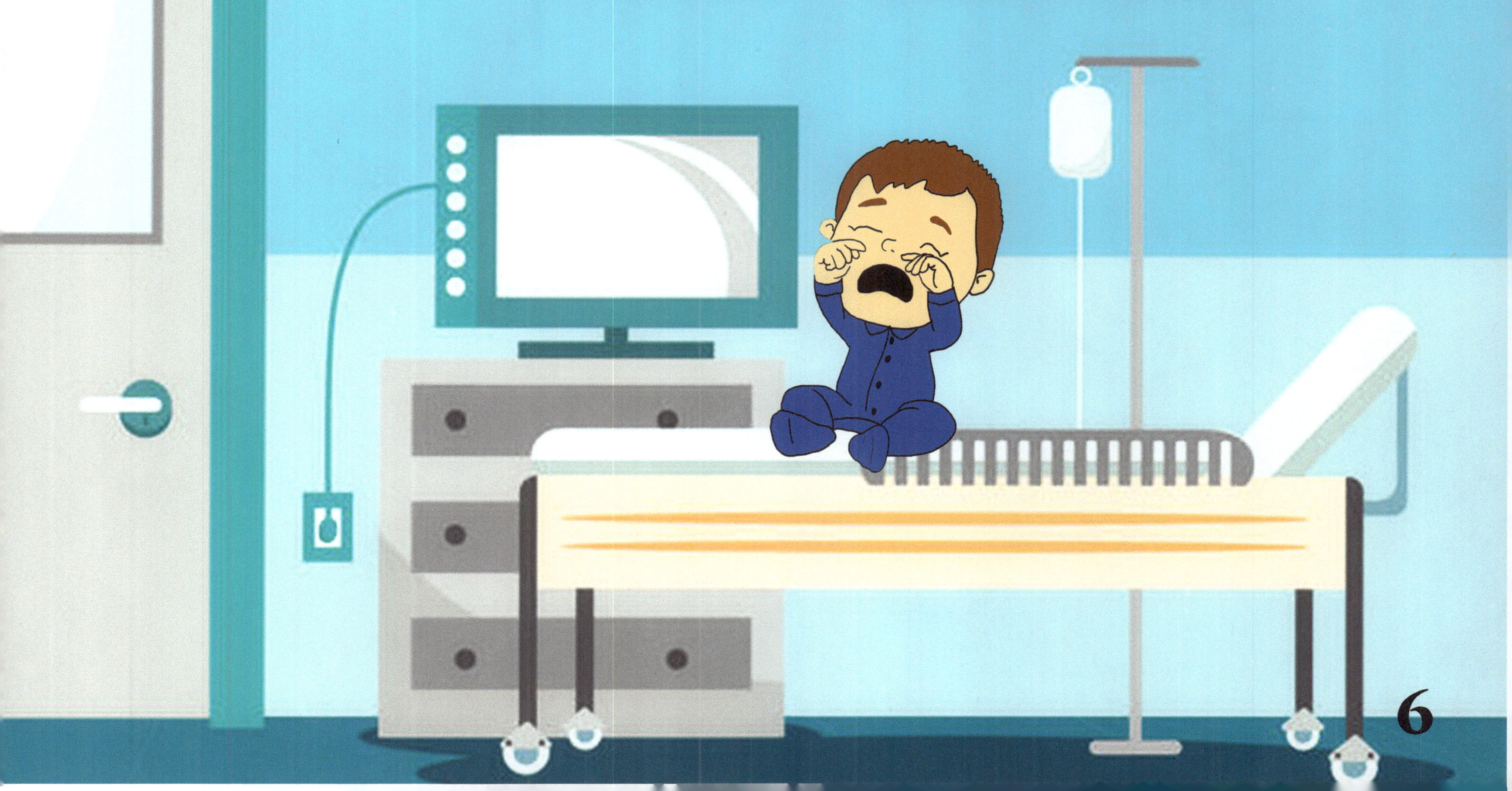

BECAUSE IT'S RARE FOR BABIES
TO GET TYPE ONE DIABETES,
IT TOOK A FEW MORE DOCTORS
TO FIND OUT
WHAT WAS HAPPENING TO ME.

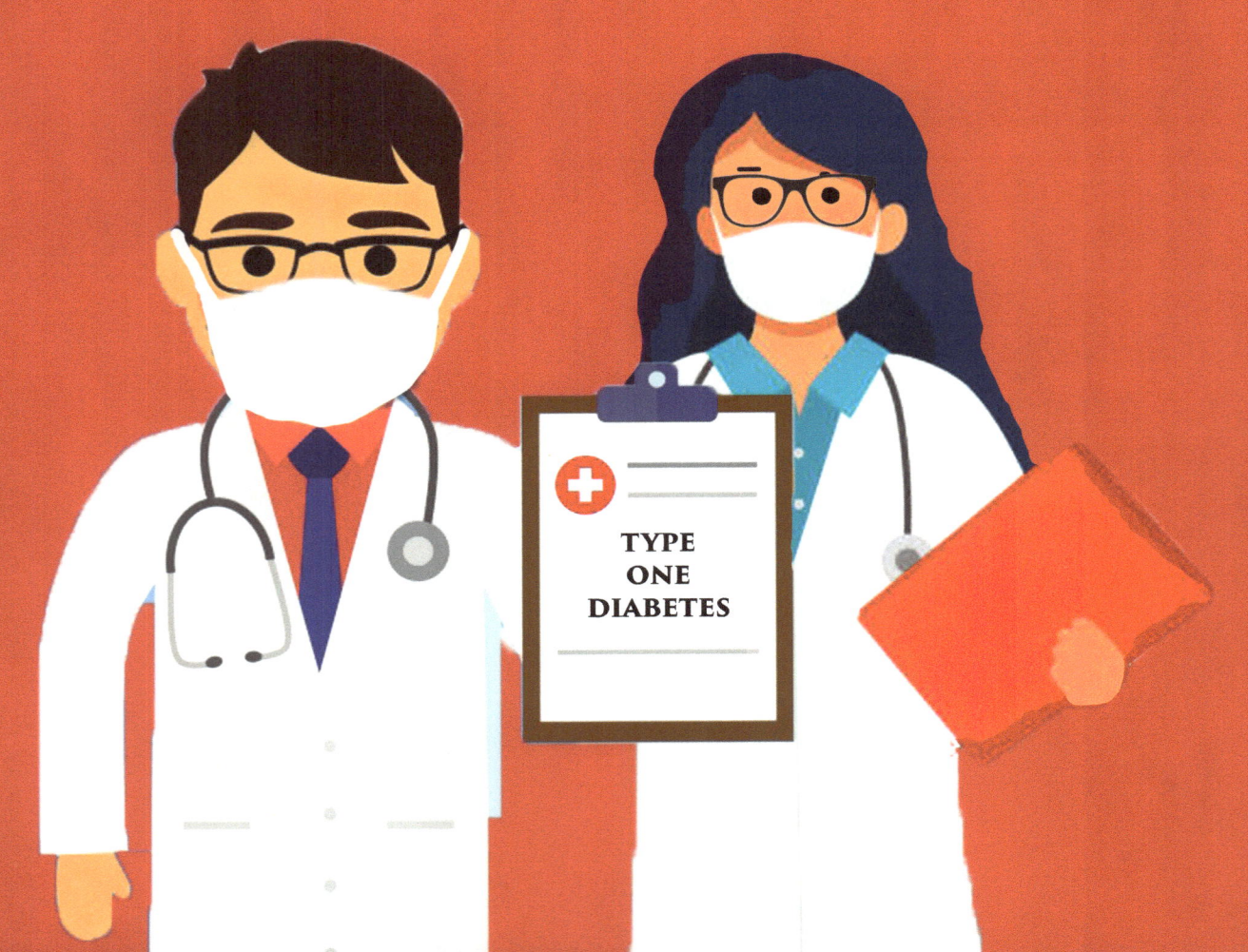

TYPE 1 DIABETES IS
AN AUTO IMMUNE DISEASE.
THERE IS NO CURE
OR PREVENTION.
MY OWN BODY ATTACKED ME.

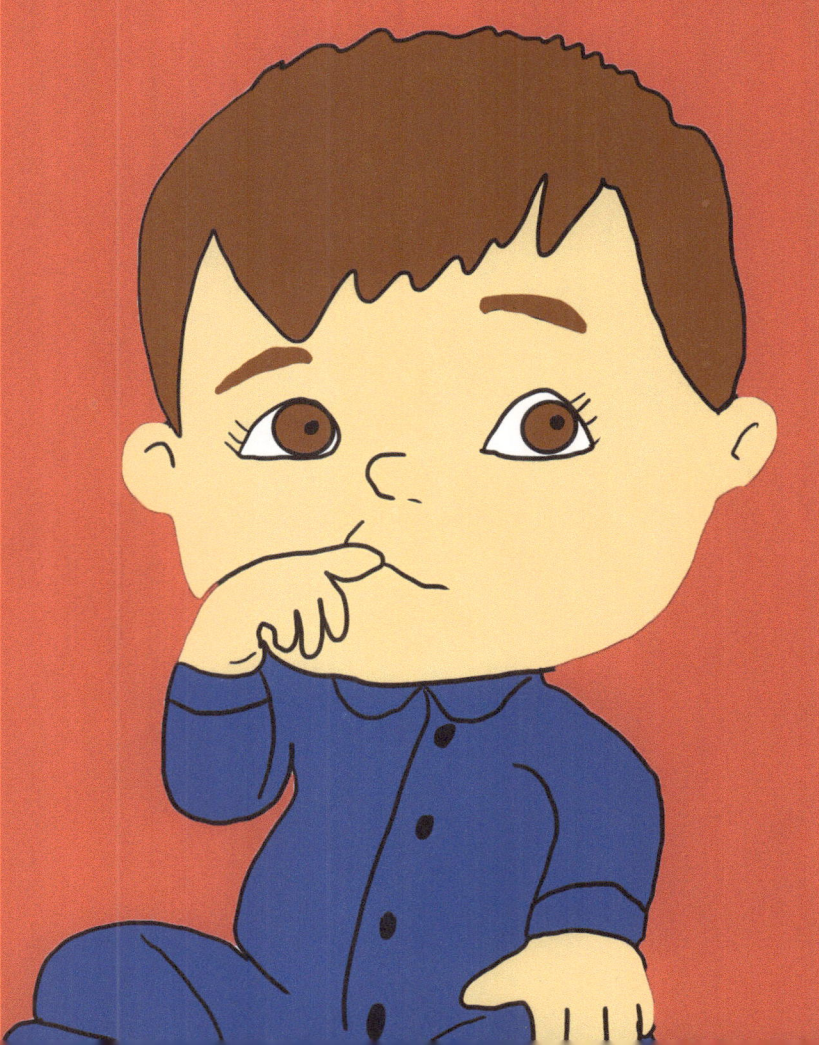

8

THE PROBLEM IS WITH MY PANCREAS, IT GOT REAL SICK ONE DAY. BECAUSE OF THIS, THE BETA CELLS WERE FORCED TO GO AWAY.

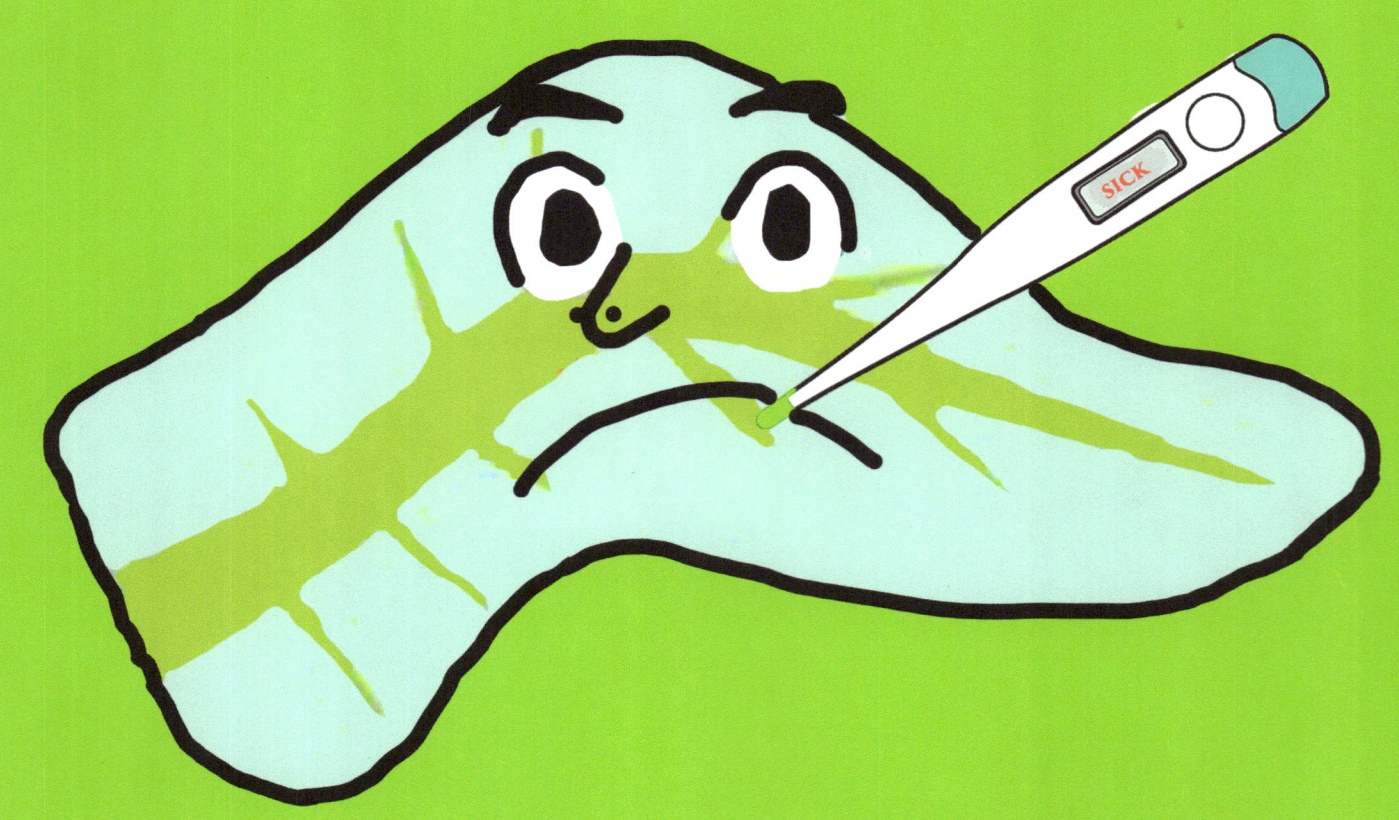

THESE CELLS PRODUCE OUR
INSULIN THAT HELP
HIGH SUGARS COME DOWN.
BUT SINCE OUR CELLS
HAVE GONE AWAY WE GET INSULIN
THROUGH NEEDLES NOW.

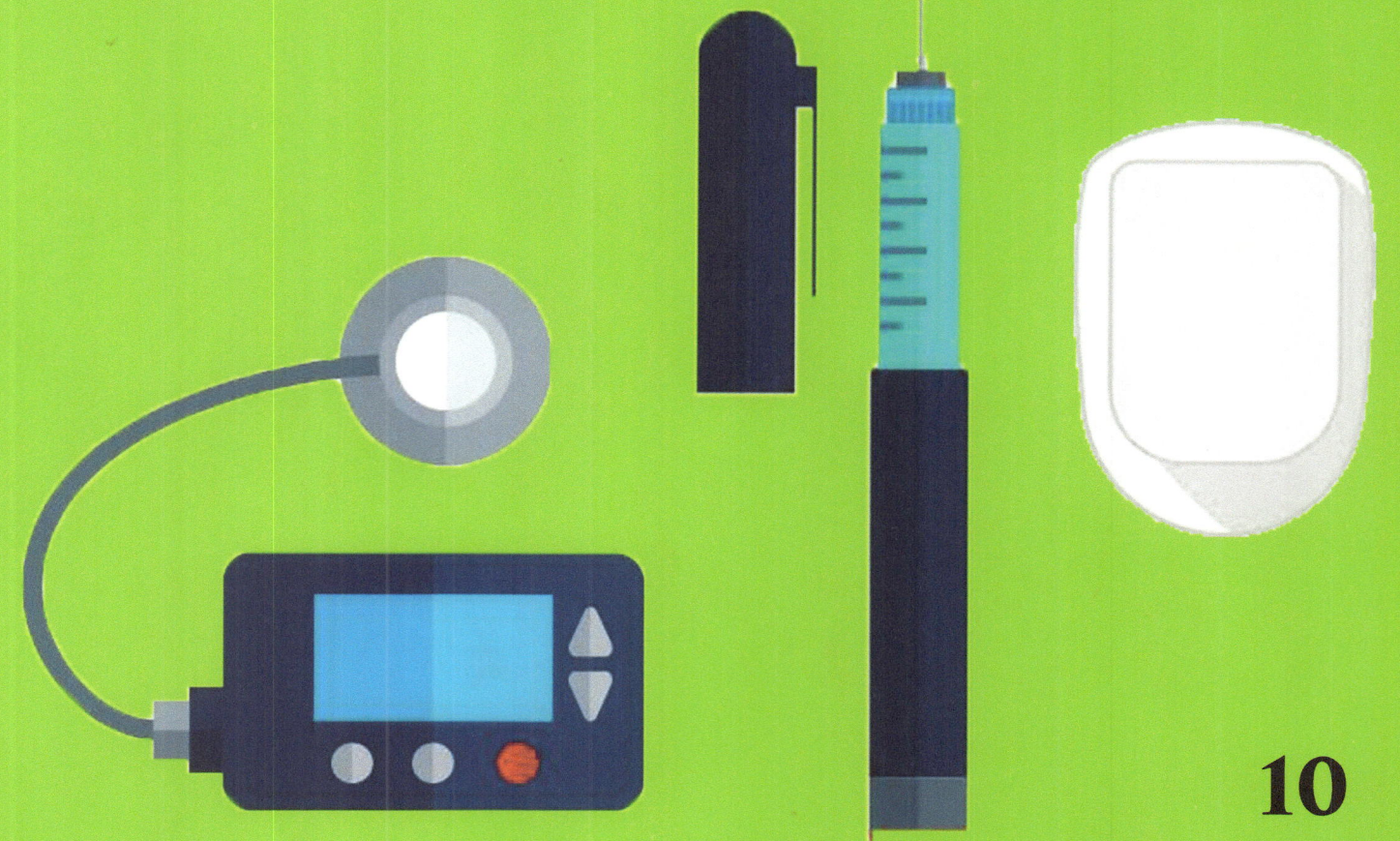

EATING HEALTHY MATTERS.
YOU WILL LOVE THE YUMMY FOOD.
YOU GET TO EAT A LOT OF MEAT
AND VEGGIES THAT ARE GOOD!

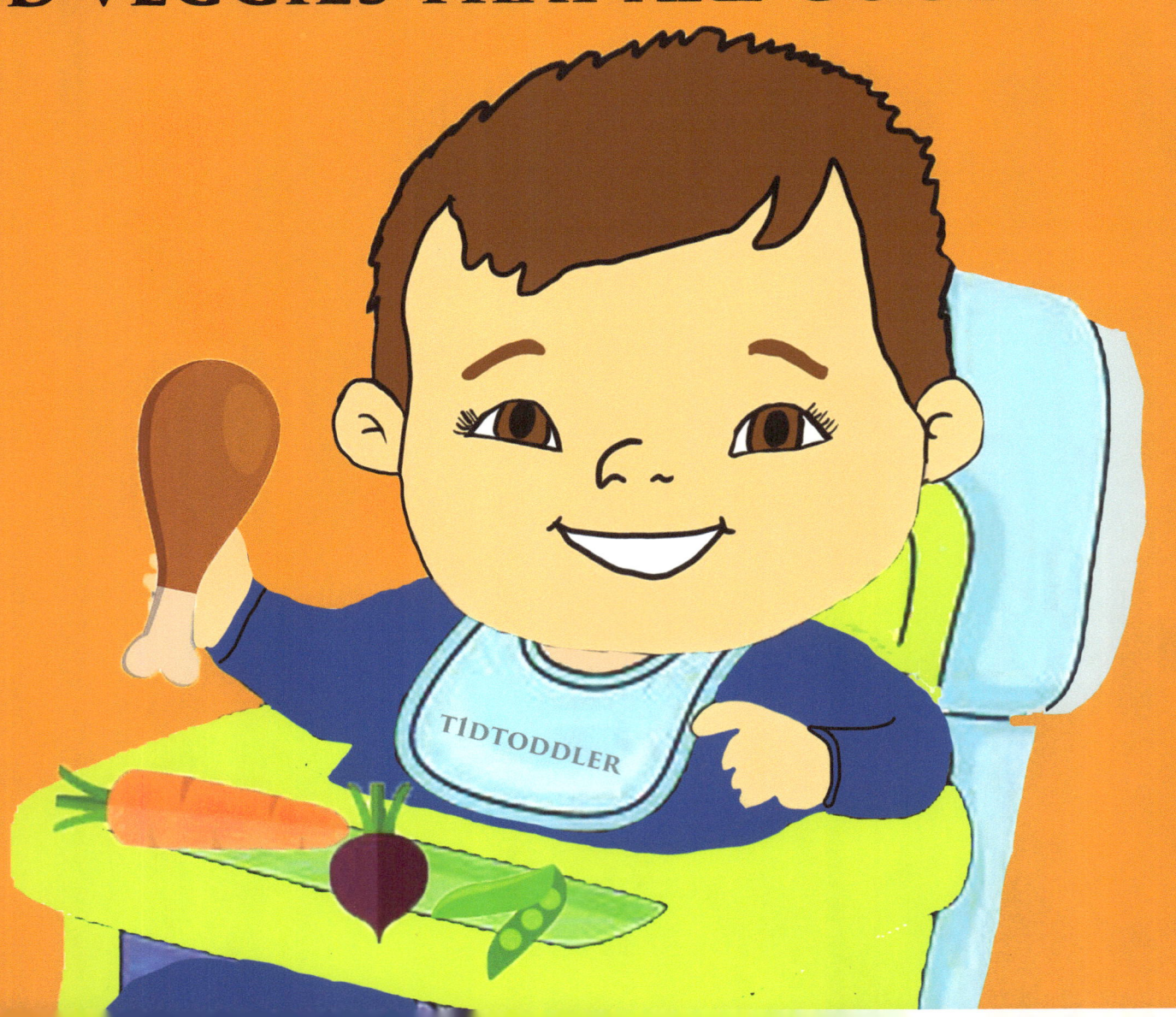

STAYING ACTIVE IS FUN.
IT'S BETTER WHEN YOU PLAY.
LAUGHING IS THE BEST,
AND YOU CAN DO THAT EVERYDAY.

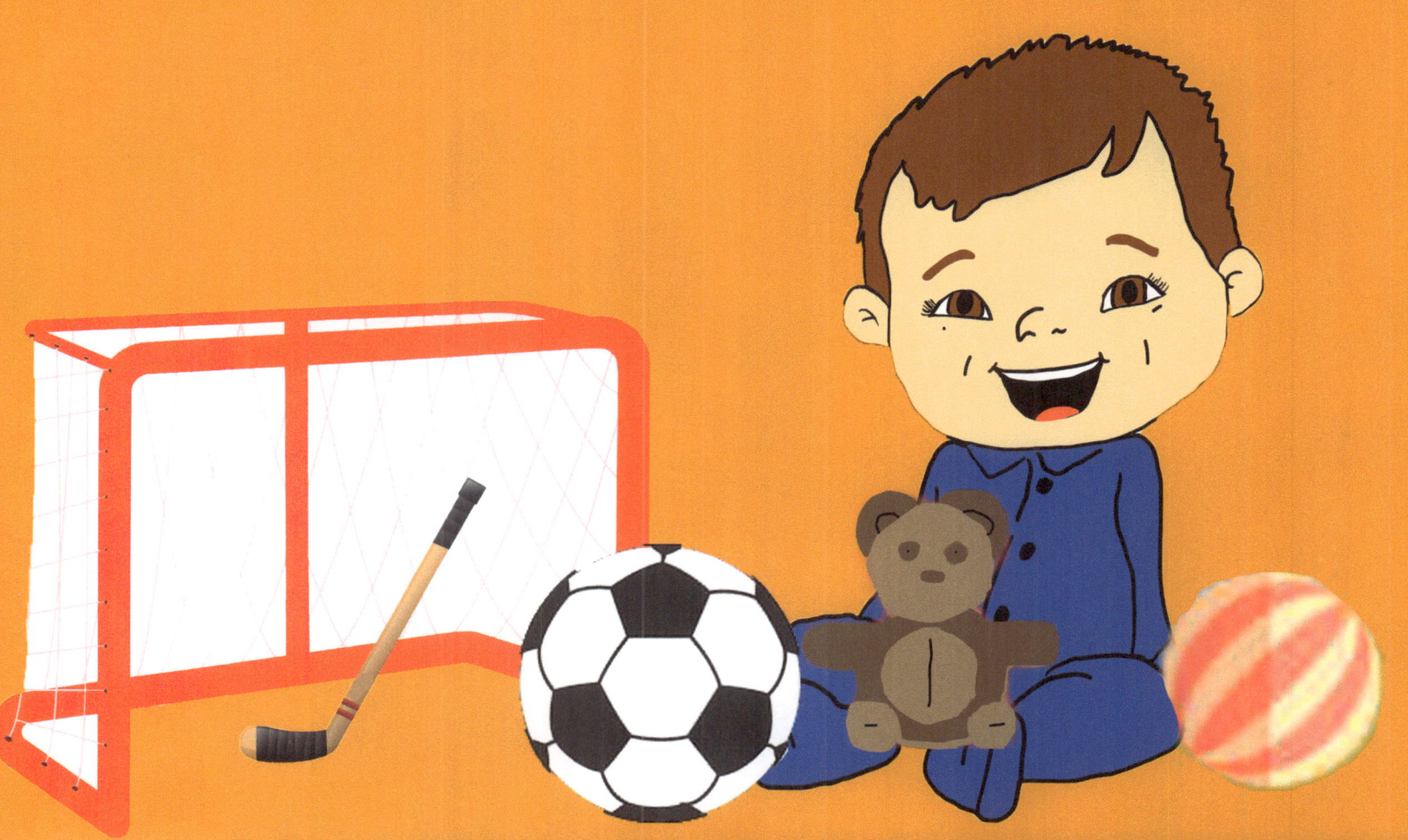

12

THE AVERAGE AGE IS OLDER AND BECAUSE WE CANNOT TALK, THE COMPLICATIONS OF DIABETES GET HIDDEN IN THE DARK.

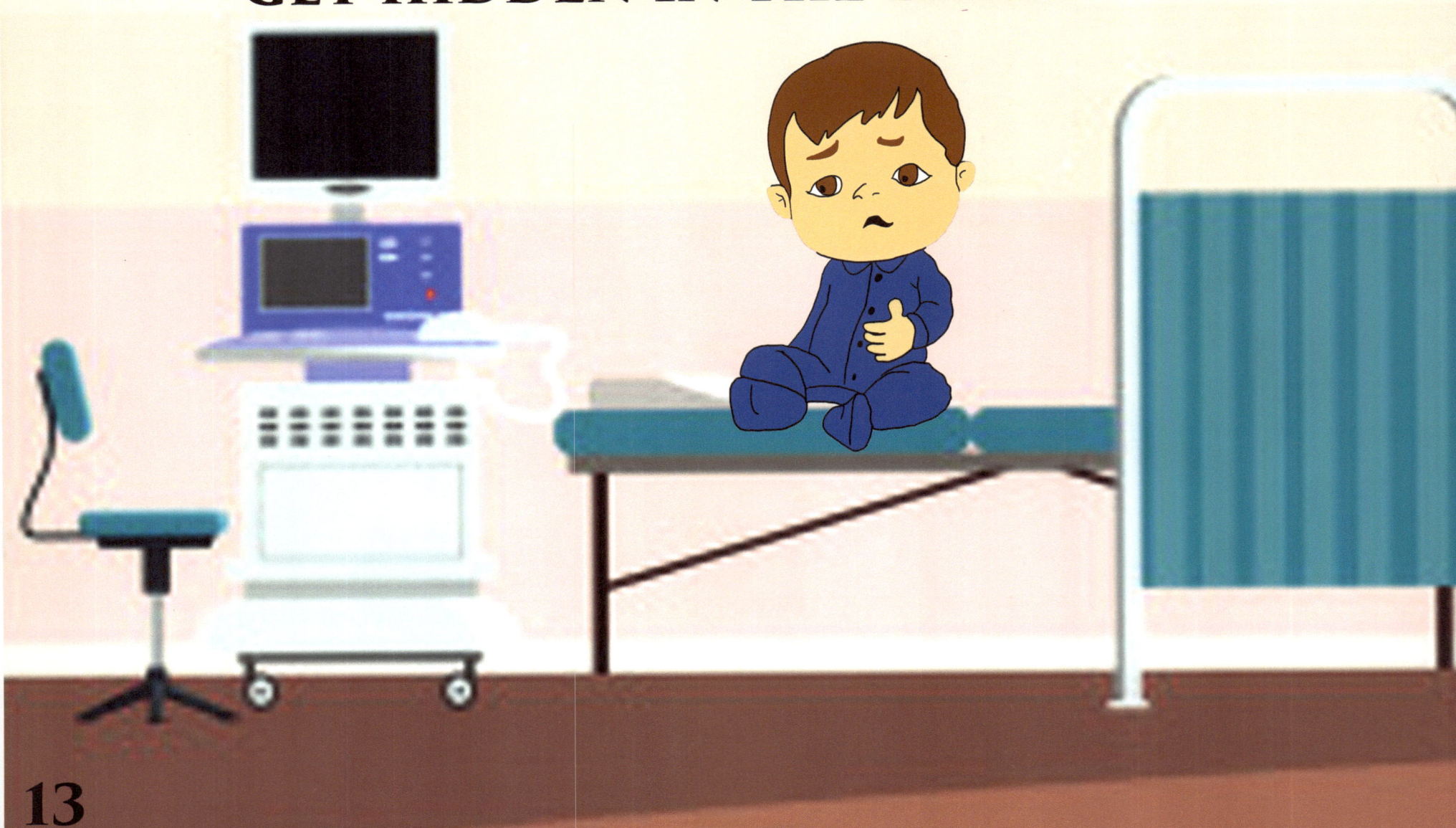

BUT LUCKILY WE HAVE HEROES,
WHO SPEAK ON OUR BEHALF.
THEY FIGHT FOR US
AND CARE FOR US,
WE CALL THEM MOM AND DAD.

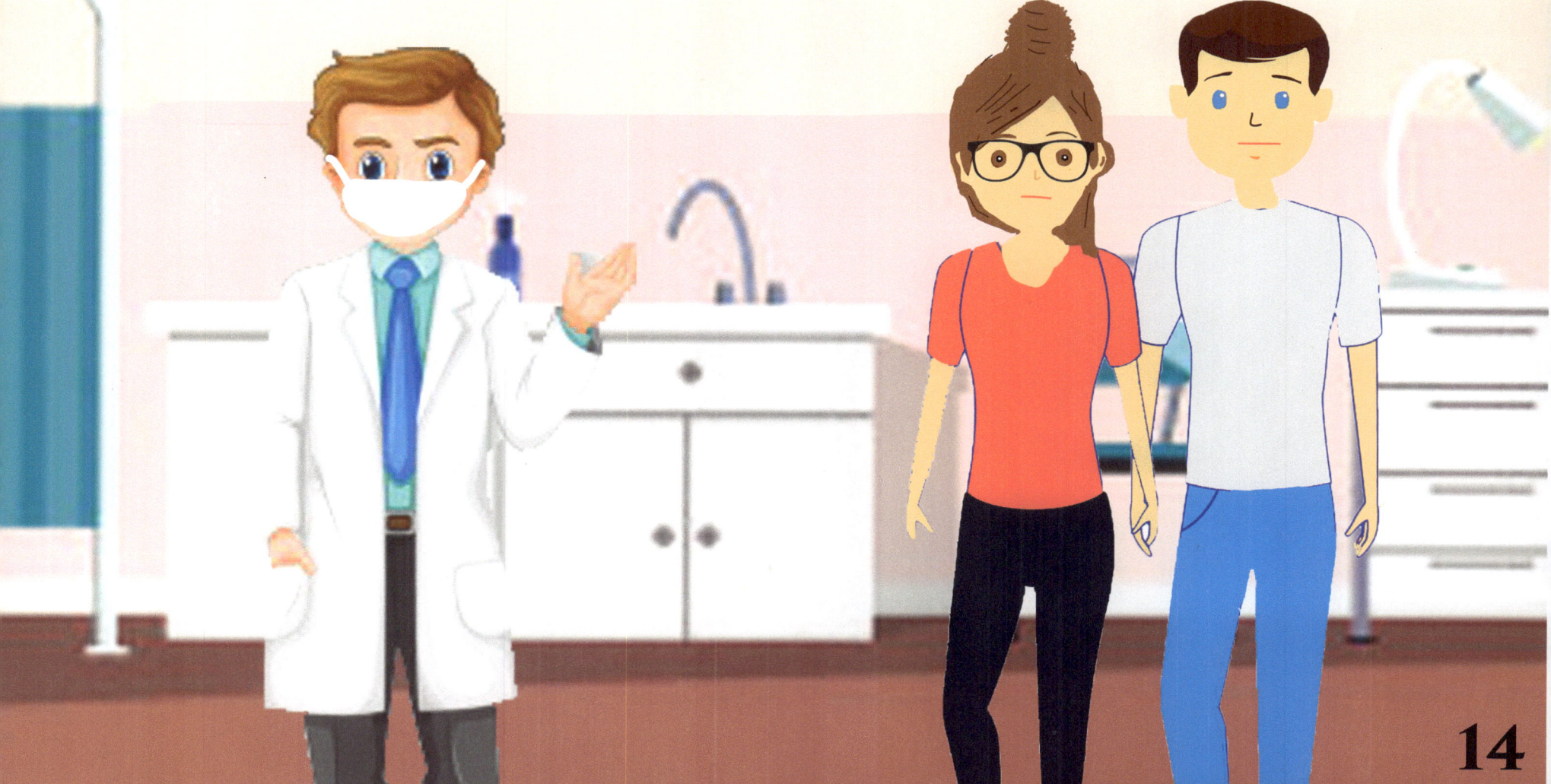

PARENTS OF T1D TODDLERS ARE ANGELS WITHOUT WINGS. THEY RESCUE US WITHOUT A DOUBT AND COMFORT ALL LIFE'S STINGS.

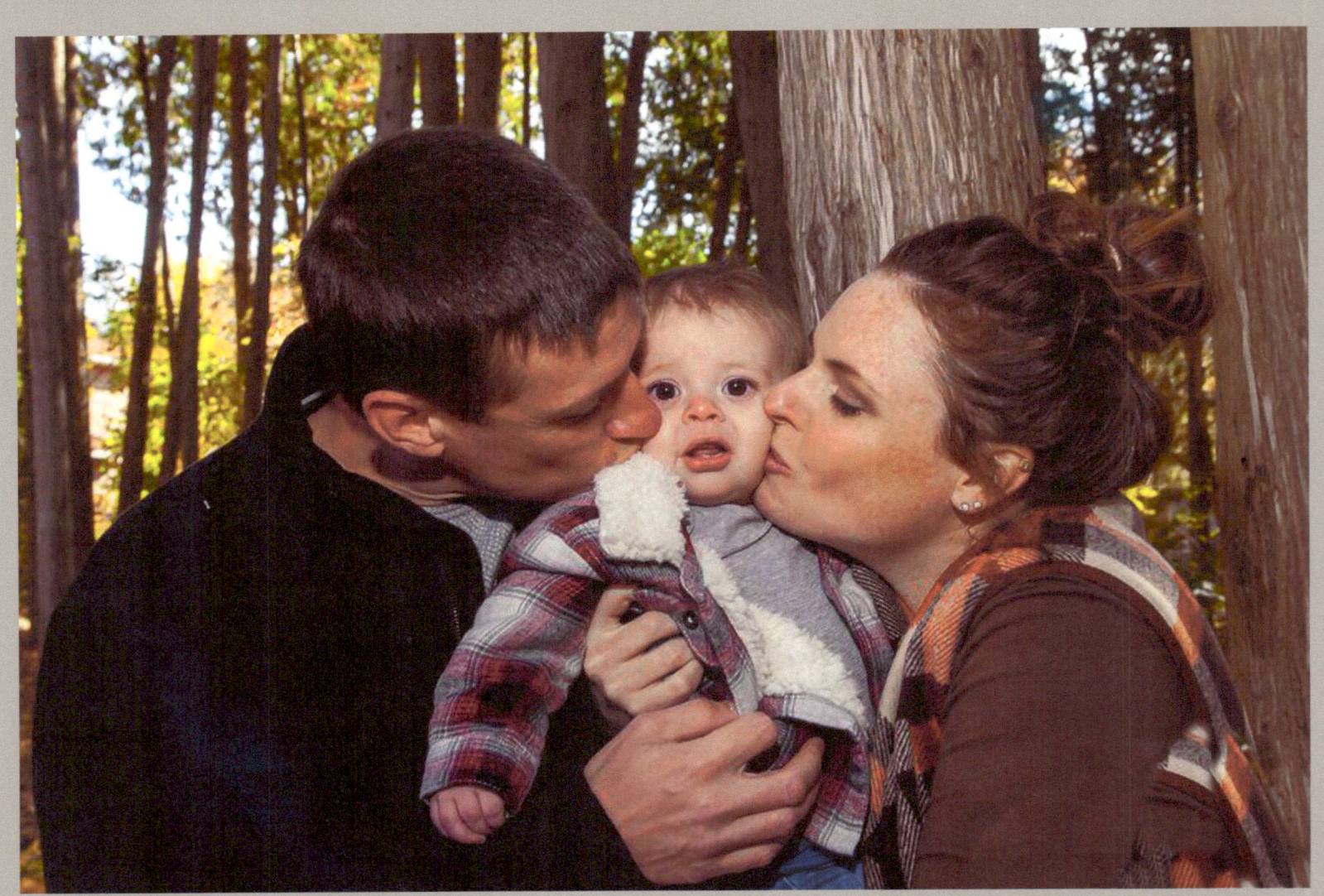

ALONG WITH OUR EQUIPMENT AND T1D COMMUNITY, SOMEDAY WE WILL FIND A CURE FOR TYPE 1 DIABETES !

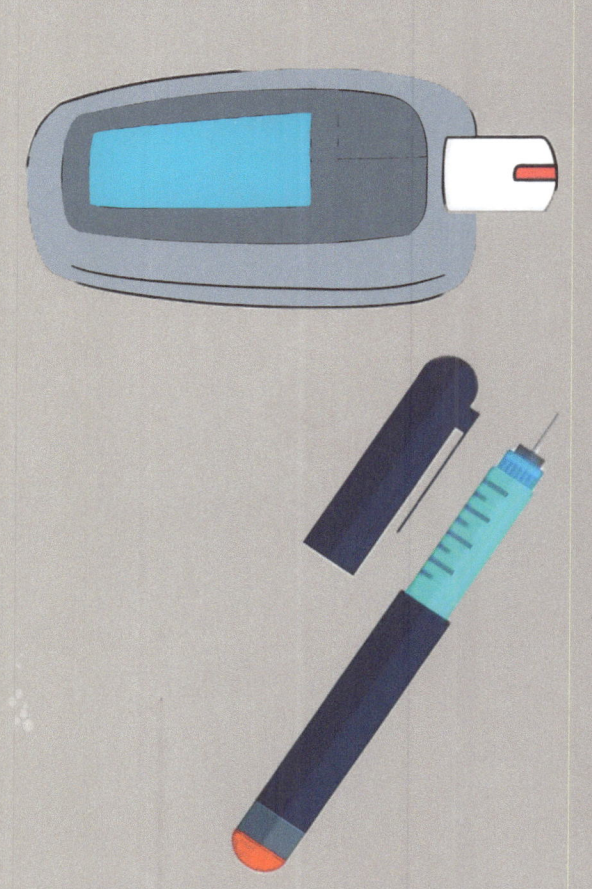

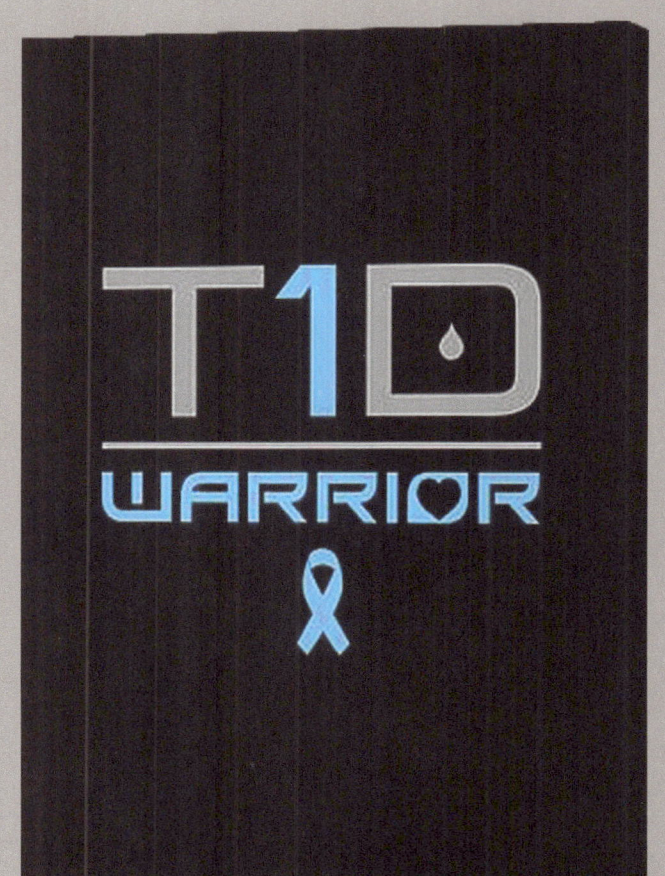

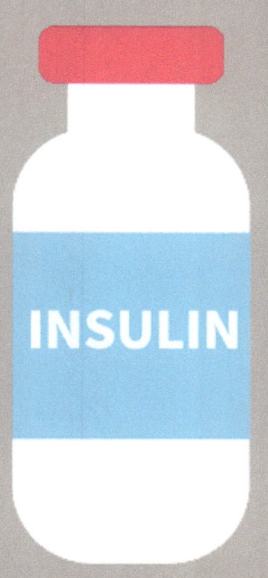

DEDICATED TO:
RYDER, SCOTT AND OUR FAMILY
ALONG WITH ALL T1D WARRIORS
AND THEIR FAMILIES.

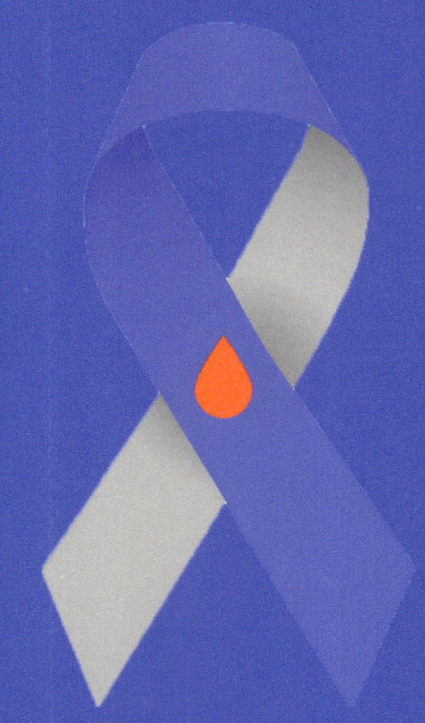

@T1DTODDLER

CPSIA information can be obtained
at www.ICGtesting.com
Printed in the USA
BVHW062113150221
600194BV00001B/9